TERFAMEX

The Complete Guide On How To Lose Weight Quickly, End Obesity Using Terfamex

Joe Amber

TERFAMEX

Terfamex is an incredibly powerful drug used for weight loss management that has quickly made its way into the mainstream market. It is a prescription medication that is typically used to treat severe obesity or to manage health risks associated with severe obesity. It is one of the newest weight loss medications to become available and it has proven to be an effective and safe treatment option for those experiencing or caring for individuals that are struggling with severe weight issues. Terfamex works by altering the hormones in the body that are related to hunger and satiety. Its main components, fenfluramine and phentermine, work in unison to control appetite, cravings, and overeating. This dual action makes it an extremely effective weight loss treatment option for individuals who are struggling with obesity and related health issues. Fenfluramine works to reduce the amount of food you consume, by blocking the reuptake of norepinephrine and serotonin from synapses in the brain. By reducing how much you eat, it helps you to reach your weight loss goals. Phentermine helps to activate your resting metabolism and increases your body's fat burning potential. This helps to expand your energy levels and reduce feelings of fatigue associated with low-calorie diets. Another important way Terfamex helps manage weight is by decreasing cravings. The medication is designed to decrease the amount of time you spend thinking about food and when you do think about food, your cravings are much weaker than before. For individuals having difficulty with overeating, this can be an incredibly beneficial tool. In order to ensure safety and effectiveness of Terfamex, it is recommended that individuals start by consulting a doctor. A physician can provide full details about the medication's safety and effectiveness and can make sure that any existing health issues do not conflict with Terfamex use. They can also recommend the best dosage for an individual's specific needs based on lifestyle, age, weight, and overall health goals. Although Terfamex is an incredibly powerful weight loss management treatment, it also comes with potential side effects that should be taken into account. These may include drowsiness, dry mouth, blurred vision, headaches, nausea, vomiting, and constipation. Additionally, some individuals may have experiences other more serious side effects such as heart valve issues or increased or decreased blood pressure. It is important to carefully consider the risks when taking Terfamex and consult your doctor if any issues arise. Terfamex is an incredibly effective weight loss management treatment when used correctly. It has been proven to be a safe and effective treatment option for individuals trying to lose weight and those managing health risks associated with obesity. By consulting a doctor and getting detailed advice on dosages and side effects, individuals will be able to take advantage of the many benefits of this medication and reduce the amount of weight gained and lost over time.

USES OF TERFAMEX

Terfamex, also known as Fenfluramine, is a medication that is used in the treatment of certain medical conditions primarily focusing on weight loss and preventing seizures. It is an anorectic, or anti-obesity medication, which has been used since the 1960s to reduce appetite and help individuals to shed excess weight. As well as its primary weight-loss purposes, Terfamex has been used to treat depression, panic attacks, obsessive-compulsive disorder (OCD) and even some forms of premenstrual dysphoric disorder (PMDD). It also has some off-label uses such as reducing the vomiting associated with chemotherapy and also for easing the symptoms of fibromyalgia. Terfamex is a type of amphetamine that belongs to the class known as catecholamines. Terfamex works by stimulating norepinephrine and serotonin in the brain. It can also bind with certain serotonin receptors in the brain, which can lead to an increase in the amount of these two chemicals. This can create a feeling of increased alertness, along with improved concentration. It has been found to be an effective appetite suppressant as well. As with many medications, there are potential side effects from taking Terfamex. Short-term side effects can include insomnia, nervousness, dizziness, headaches, restlessness and dry mouth. Individuals who take this medication for a longer duration may experience an increased risk of stroke or cardiac arrest. It is also not recommended for pregnant or breastfeeding women, or those with a family history of heart disease or stroke. Due to its active ingredients, Terfamex can interact with other medications as well. They can reduce the effects of antidepressants, antipsychotics, and certain other medications if they are taken together. Since it can also interact with certain herbal supplements, it is important to discuss any medications or supplements that one is currently taking with their healthcare provider before beginning Terfamex. While Terfamex is primarily marketed as a weight-loss medication, it can be utilized in many different ways and individuals should speak to their healthcare provider to determine the best way to use it for their specific circumstances. As with any drug, it is important to take it exactly as prescribed and not to take it in combination with any other medications or supplements. Taking it as prescribed should help to reduce any potential side effects and increase its effectiveness.

DOSING INFORMATION

Terfamex is a brand name for a drug compound of venlafaxine and mexiletine. Venlafaxine is a serotonin-noradrenaline reuptake inhibitor (SNRI) antidepressant, while mexiletine is an antiarrhythmic used to treat irregular heart rhythms. It is available in capsule form and used to treat major depressive disorder and generalized anxiety disorder in adults. Due to its ability to alter both serotonin and noradrenaline levels in the brain, Terfamex targets both the physical and psychological symptoms associated with depression. It works by inhibiting the uptake of neurotransmitters in the brain, allowing more of these chemicals to circulate in the brain and have a beneficial effect on mood and behavior. The recommended daily dosage of Terfamex for adults is between 75 to 225 mg per day taken in divided doses. It is usually started at a low dose of 37.5 mg per day for 7 to 14 days before increasing to the recommended range of 75 to 225 mg per day. Dosages higher than 225 mg a day have not been proven to be effective so should be avoided. When taken in the form of extended-release capsules, it should be taken with food or immediately after a meal to reduce possible adverse effects. It should not be chewed or crushed as this could result in an unintended release of medication into the bloodstream. It is important to follow the recommended dosage instructions provided by your doctor or pharmacist and take it regularly as directed. You may experience an improvement in mood within two to four weeks of starting therapy, however, it may take several months to experience the full benefits of using this drug. It is possible to experience side effects with using Terfamex. Common side effects include difficulty sleeping, nausea, headaches, increased sweating, and anxiety. These side effects are usually mild and tend to lessen or go away with time. More severe side effects such as irregular heartbeat, difficulty breathing, and decreased white blood cells in the blood have also been reported. If you experience any of these side effects, contact your doctor immediately. If you miss a dose, it is important to take it as soon as you remember. Do not take an extra dose to make up for the missed dose. Doing so may result in a sudden increase in the amount of medication in your body, which could result in an overdose. Stopping treatment suddenly is not advised as this could result in withdrawal symptoms, such as drowsiness, nausea, vomiting, dizziness, and tiredness. If you are considering stopping your treatment, it is important to speak to your doctor about slowly weaning yourself off the drug. The safety and efficacy of using this drug in pregnant or breastfeeding women has not been established. Patients should consult with their doctor before taking Terfamex if they are pregnant, planning to become pregnant, or breastfeeding. Due to its effects on the brain, Terfamex should not be taken with certain types of drugs, such as MAOIs, alprazolam, St. John's wort, or bupropion. Patients should consult their doctor or pharmacist before taking Terfamex with any other medication to ensure it is safe to do so. Terfamex is a SNRI antidepressant used to treat major depressive disorder and generalized anxiety disorder in adults. It is important to strictly adhere to the recommended dosage instructions and should not be taken with certain types of drugs. If you experience any side effects or are considering stopping treatment, consult your doctor.

SIDE EFFECTS

The side effects of Terfamex can be numerous and potentially dangerous for those who take the drug. Terfamex is a brand name of phentermine, a weight-loss drug recently approved by the U.S. Food and Drug Administration for short-term use. People typically take it by mouth, often in pill or capsule form. While the drug can help some individuals shed pounds, it also carries risks and potential side effects that should be taken into consideration before taking the drug. Common side effects of Terfamex include increased heart rate, increased blood pressure, anxiety, insomnia, nausea, constipation, headaches, dry mouth, diarrhea, increased sweating, and blurred vision. Short-term use of Terfamex may also lead to changes in mood and behavior, including restlessness, irritability, and depression. Some side effects are more serious than others, with some being potentially dangerous for those who take the drug. These more serious side effects can include pulmonary hypertension (high blood pressure in the lungs), heart valve diseases, stroke, and even heart attack. Long-term use of Terfamex can also increase the person's risk for developing serious cardiovascular problems, such as high blood pressure or heart failure. People taking the drug should therefore be closely monitored, as even short-term use may result in serious side effects. In addition, long-term use of Terfamex may lead to a phenomenon known as weight cycling, or yo-yo dieting, where the person experiences rapid weight gain after stopping the drug. This may be due to the body trying to compensate for the drop in energy that results from the changes in appetite caused by Terfamex. In addition to these common side effects, there are some other, more rare issues that have been reported in those taking Terfamex. These include decreased libido and impotence, increased aggression and hostility, confusion, hallucinations, memory loss, and even psychosis. Terfamex has also been found to be linked to addiction and dependence in some people. Individuals should speak to a professional about these risks before taking the drug. Terfamex can be an effective method for weight loss, but it should be taken seriously. Side effects of Terfamex can potentially be very severe, even in those taking the drug in the short term. Even individuals taking the drug for long-term use should be aware of potential risks and side effects so that they can make an informed decision. Additionally, for those struggling with addiction and dependence, seeking professional help is the best solution for their safety.

HOW TO TAKE TERFAMEX

When it comes to taking terfamex, it's important to take the time to understand how it works and what precautions to take. Terfamex is a drug commonly used to treat pain, especially in people with chronic inflammatory conditions like rheumatoid arthritis or other joint diseases. This drug has some powerful effects, so it's important to familiarize yourself with any potential risks and side effects it may have. The first step for anyone looking to take terfamex should be to talk to their doctor. In most cases, a doctor will assess a patient's individual needs and medical history and determine if terfamex is suitable to take. If the drug is deemed appropriate, the patient should receive a prescription and instructions on how to take the medication. The recommended dosage of terfamex will depend on the patient and the condition being treated. A patient's age, weight, and other factors also need to be taken into consideration. This means that a patient may be prescribed a different strength or frequency. Never change the prescribed dosage or frequency without consulting a healthcare professional first. Terfamex should be taken exactly as instructed by a doctor. In most cases, the medication is taken orally and with a full glass of water (at least 8 ounces). It's also important to take terfamex with food, as it can cause an upset stomach. When taking the medication, it is important to swallow it whole and not chew or crush the tablets. Given terfamex's powerful effects, it is important to be aware of any potential side effects. Common side effects include nausea, dizziness, and constipation. If a patient experiences any side effects, they should speak to a doctor immediately. There are also a number of serious side effects associated with terfamex, such as serious skin rashes, vision changes, muscle weakness, confusion, and breathing difficulties. For anyone taking terfamex, it's important not to stop taking the medication abruptly. Suddenly stopping can cause a number of unpleasant withdrawal symptoms. In most cases, a doctor will gradually taper a patient off the medication in a safe and controlled way to limit any potential withdrawal effects. When taking terfamex, it's important to have regular appointments with a doctor to monitor the effect the drug is having on the patient's condition. During these appointments, the patient should inform the doctor of any side effects or concerns they have about the drug. In some cases, the doctor may prefer the patient to have regular blood tests to check the drug's concentration in the blood. Taking terfamex can be a powerful and effective way to manage pain in some conditions, but it's important to follow the instructions of a healthcare professional. Knowing the risks associated with the drug and being aware of any side effects will help ensure terfamex is taken safely and effectively.

Made in the USA
Coppell, TX
10 December 2023